Preface

Keto and Intermittent Fasting — the latest buzz in the world of dieting. With so much information (and misinformation) floating around online, it's no wonder people are overwhelmed and unsure where to start.

We tend to give this "diet craze" only half the credit it deserves. But the truth is, it's simple, effective, and adaptable — you can make it work for your lifestyle, no matter where you are.

The Keto Experiment isn't your typical step-by-step guide filled with strict meal plans, complex recipes, and overwhelming measurements. Instead, it's a motivational resource designed to help *anyone* succeed. You'll find tools, encouragement, and real-life insights to support your journey.

Now, let me be honest — I'm not a professional author. So, read this with an open heart. When I asked friends how to start, they told me, "Write like you're talking to someone you care about." And if you know me, you know I'm country — but I did just that anyway.

Writing this book was more than just sharing a diet. It became a form of therapy — a way to heal from poor self-image, low self-esteem, and the health struggles I'd been battling. It's also my way of giving back: by helping others take that first step toward feeling better inside and out.

So before you dive in, take a moment. Ask yourself why this book found its way into your hands. What are you looking for? What are you ready to take back control of?

Your journey to better physical and mental health starts here — and I'll be cheering you on every step of the way. Visit my blog at https://samarahardee.blogspot.com. Share your wins, ask questions, and let's keep pushing toward your Keto success — together.

Index

Dedication:

This book is dedicated to my three children, Reese, Chess, and Gabby whom I love and adore with all my heart. May they see their worth and work towards great things and happiness, learn from my mistakes, and grow from their own.

"Failure is merely practice in motion." Andy Frisella

Love,
Mom

Introduction

Hey there, friend! If you're anything like me, you've tried **EVERY** diet in the book (and probably stared longingly at the cookie jar a few times, too). For years I hopped from one fad diet to the next—low-fat, no carbs, crazy juice cleanses—you name it. I'd lose a few pounds, feel excited for a minute... and then *bam*, the weight would sneak back on. I felt stuck, frustrated, and honestly a bit hopeless at times.

Then one day, almost by accident, I discovered something that literally changed the game: **keto and intermittent fasting**. Yep, two words that totally terrified me at first (I mean, me eating FAT to lose fat?!). But curiosity got the best of me. I dove into YouTube rabbit holes and blog posts late into the night, and the more I learned, the more excited I got.

I'll never forget the day it finally clicked: I was tired of feeling tired, and I was ready to try something **REAL**. I gave keto a shot, cutting out sugar and carbs and loading up on butter, avocado, and bacon (yes, *bacon!*). I paired it with intermittent fasting—just giving my body longer breaks between meals—and something incredible happened. The scale started moving, slowly at first, then faster. Week by week, I saw results: no more mid-afternoon crashes, pants feeling looser, and a spark of confidence.

Honestly, I never thought I'd say these words... but I **LOVED** those transformations! I was running (jogging? Okay, *very determined walking* counts!) in the morning, bursting with clarity during the day, and sleeping like a LOG at night. Friends and family noticed the change; strangers asked if I was the same person. This wasn't just weight melting off—it was me *coming back to life.* Every day felt like a tiny victory. Heck, I even stuck a note on my fridge saying *Progress, not perfection.* It became my mantra whenever I needed a reminder.

Look, I totally get how overwhelming this can be. You might feel like I did: skeptical, worried, maybe a little scared to try yet another "diet of the month." But listen: *you are not alone*, and **YOU CAN DO THIS**. I wrote this little book for you because I wish someone had handed *me* all these tips, tricks, and lessons in one place. No fluff—just honest talk about what worked, what didn't, and how I kept myself motivated when I wanted to quit.

Now, before we dive into the real meat of this book, here are some **VIDEO RECOMMENDATIONS** that fired me up and taught me a lot. Check these out when you need inspiration or a quick keto/IF how-to:

- *Keto for Beginners* – A friendly YouTube intro to how keto works (I watched this the first night I decided, "Okay, I'm actually going to try this!").

- *My 100-Pound Weight Loss on Keto and Fasting* – An inspiring transformation story. Seeing someone else do it made me realize I could too.

- *Why Intermittent Fasting Matters* – A motivating talk (or video) that explains the science behind fasting without putting you to sleep. Totally changed the way I see meal times.

That's my story in a nutshell—an honest, messy, excited account of how keto and IF turned my life around. I promise, if I can do it (and I was *that* person who never stuck to a diet!), then you can absolutely do it too. So grab your favorite coffee (or tea), settle in, and let's get started on **YOUR** journey. **YOU'VE GOT THIS!**

Chapter 1: My Journey – Where It All Began

Like most kids, my story started out pretty normal. I was born to two very young parents, in a modest three-bedroom house on a dusty backroad somewhere in middle-west Georgia. I had an older sister, lots of cousins nearby, and even a dog. Life was simple... for a while.

Back then, I was a healthy, average-sized kid. But things started to change when my parents' relationship fell apart. The fights, the yelling, the tension—it created a kind of storm inside our home. I was too young to understand it all, but I felt every bit of the stress. Their divorce wasn't just sad, it was violent and chaotic. At one point, things got so bad that my sister and I were almost put into foster care.

Thank God for my grandmother. She stepped in and took us under her wing. During kindergarten and first grade, we lived with her. My mom would sneak visits when she could, always careful because my father had made some serious threats. She'd wait until he left for work, then take the back roads to come see us. Looking back, that time with my grandmother was one of the safest, most comforting periods of my childhood.

Eventually, the court gave custody to my mom. That meant we had to move in with her and her boyfriend—away from the wide-open spaces of my grandmother's home and into a cramped Atlanta apartment. It was cleaner and safer than some places, but it never felt like *home*. My sister and I were latchkey kids. We came home to an empty apartment after school and stayed locked inside until our mom got home from work. We didn't run outside or play in the dirt anymore—we just sat.

The home-cooked, healthy meals from the garden were replaced with fast food, TV dinners, and convenience store snacks. I remember grabbing a Zinger and a Coke from the 7-Eleven on school mornings—that was breakfast. That's how the unhealthy habits started.

The less we moved, the more we ate. Out of boredom, out of comfort, out of stress. And where was my dad during all this? After a huge blowup between him and my mom—guns, screaming, the whole terrifying scene—he basically vanished. My sister and I spent summers with our grandmother and aunt instead. No complaints there—that was the best part of my childhood.

But by middle school, my weight was no longer something I could ignore. My mom tried. She really did. She put me in weight loss programs, bought the diet sodas, signed me up for Weight Watchers, low-fat everything—you name it. Nothing worked.

Then came the hypnotist. Yep, at just 13 years old and weighing 148 pounds, my mom took me to someone who claimed to help people lose weight through hypnosis. And you know what? That year, I lost 50 pounds. Maybe it was the hypnosis. Maybe I just hit a breaking point. But for the first time, I saw results—and I liked the attention it brought.

After that, I moved in with my dad, his new wife, and their baby. That came with its own set of challenges. My dad wasn't exactly welcoming. He joked about my weight, left me out of things, and made me feel like I didn't belong. But I kept the weight off for a while—through most of high school, I stayed under 130 pounds.

But then... I got into a relationship with a man who was way too old for me. I was just 15, and he was 24. I was in way over my head. That relationship chipped away at my self-esteem, and slowly, the weight crept back on. I tried everything to fight it: running, walking, dieting, restricting. Nothing worked for long.

And that was just the start of my lifelong battle with weight.

Over the years, I tried every diet under the sun. Atkins, Jenny Craig, Protein Power, South Beach, Paleo, Whole30, you name it. I drank the shakes, popped the pills (prescription and over-the-counter), combined foods in weird ways, even did that ridiculous three-day diet where you get to eat ice cream. But no matter what I did, I could never lose the stubborn fat around my belly, arms, and thighs.

Doctors kept giving me the same advice: count calories, cut fat, watch sugar. I followed it all, but the weight stayed. Each failed attempt left me feeling more defeated than the last.

Then came my thirties. I met a tall, handsome man, and within two months we were living together and expecting our first child. I worked full-time, cooked big family meals, tried to be the perfect wife and mother. But during pregnancy, I was diagnosed with gestational diabetes and ballooned to 225 pounds. After giving birth, I was exhausted, overwhelmed, and absolutely miserable in my own skin.

Not long after, I got pregnant again—this time with my son, who would later be diagnosed with severe allergies. I spent countless sleepless nights rocking and holding him as he cried in discomfort. With no energy, I turned to food for comfort and fuel. And the weight piled on.

By the time I had my third child, I was over 250 pounds.

Then something shifted.

A new public track opened up near our home, and the very first day it opened, I laced up my shoes and ran a mile. That mile turned into many. I dropped 80 pounds and finally got under 200. I felt good—better than I had in years. But still, no matter how hard I worked, that belly fat, those arms, and thighs—they just wouldn't budge.

Ten years passed. My marriage hit a rough patch. Depression crept in. While my husband worked on his abs, I was stuck in survival mode, living off snacks and stress. I reached 209 pounds again and felt completely lost.

Then, in college, I took a Healthy Lifestyle class. We had to do a health assessment. My numbers were bad—high blood pressure, high LDL, pre-diabetic. Combine that with my family history, and it was like staring down the barrel of a heart attack or stroke. I had young kids who needed me. That was my wake-up call.

I used a workplace weight-loss challenge to jumpstart my journey. But here's the kicker—I had no plan. I didn't follow a program or sign up for another weight-loss gimmick. I just decided: *I'm done failing. It's time to figure out what actually works for me.*

And not having a plan? That was the beginning of everything changing.

Chapter 2: Mindset is Everything

Let me be real with you—2018 hit me hard.

My marriage was struggling. My mindset was worse. Juggling full-time motherhood, a job in public school education, and college classes was grinding me down. I was exhausted. I was discouraged. I felt like I was drowning in expectations—with no time or energy left for me.

But then, I decided it was time to fight back.

I kicked off the year with a challenge I started at work called "Weight Down." We each chipped in $15–20 to join, and the goal was simple: lose the most weight by the end of April. If you gained a pound, you owed $2. I needed something—anything—to motivate me. And oh, I was MOTIVATED. I was angry. I was tired. I was fed up and DONE feeling like crap. Life had punched me in the gut, and I was swinging back.

That's when Keto crashed into my life. Right there on my social media feed, it popped up like a sign from above. I didn't just dabble—I researched the heck out of it. My college education kicked in. I knew how to dig deep, read the real sources, and understand the science. And what I found made sense.

I wasn't just fat—I was furious. Furious with myself. Furious at how people looked at me. Furious about the way my spouse treated me. I blamed my weight for my emotional mess, my fatigue, my mood swings, and my health. My body hurt. My hair was falling out. Wrinkles were forming, and I couldn't recognize myself in the mirror. I was pre-diabetic, depressed, and spiraling.

So I screamed. I cried. I sat in silence. And then I got to work.

Like Billy Alsbrooks says, I used all of that pain as lighter fluid. It was time to ignite something new.

And now I ask you—are YOU ready?

Are you tired of hiding in pictures? Tired of tugging on shirts to cover the rolls? Tired of your spouse acting differently toward you? Tired of being too tired to live?

Get real. Get raw. Get mad if you have to. Then use that fire to start something that could change your life.

Let me remind you—YOU ARE WORTH IT. Not just kind of. Not someday. Not if you lose 20 pounds. Right now.

Chapter 3: What Is Keto?

Let me clear this up right now:

KETO IS NOT A DIET.
 It's a Way of Eating (WOE)—a lifestyle shift, not a short-term fix. Keto is a mindset. A commitment. A daily reminder that your health and happiness are worth fighting for.

So What *Is* Keto?

Back in 1921, Dr. Russel Wilder coined the term "ketogenic diet" to treat children with epilepsy. It wasn't about weight loss—it was about healing the brain and body. Fast forward a few decades, and Keto reemerged as a powerful tool for fat loss and metabolic health.

Here's the basic breakdown:

- High fat (about 60%)
- Moderate protein (30%)
- Very low carbs (5–10%)—no sugar

To stay in ketosis, your daily carbs should stay under 20g (max 50g). That's it.

How It Works:

Normally, your body uses carbs (glucose) for energy. But when you stop feeding it carbs, your insulin levels drop, and your body enters ketosis—a fat-burning mode where it starts using ketones (made from fat) as fuel.

In other words: You burn fat instead of sugar.
 Stored fat. Belly fat. Waistline fat. That stubborn, frustrating fat.

Think about it: Diabetes, heart disease, and metabolic issues often center around belly fat. Keto helps shrink that.

If your waist is over 35 inches (women) or 40 inches (men), your risk for serious disease skyrockets (National Heart, Lung, and Blood Institute, 2018). But Keto can change that. It changed mine.

Chapter 4: What Makes Keto Easy

Keto didn't just help me lose weight—it gave me my life back. But first, I had to change my mindset.

I started this journey MAD at myself. But anger was just the match—I needed fuel. And fuel came in the form of truth. I had to forgive myself. For the weight. The poor choices. The self-neglect. The broken relationships. All of it.

I didn't need a therapist (though nothing wrong if you do)—I needed a plan.

In college, I created a wellness project and evaluated my health risks. Stress, anxiety, emotional eating. My family history was a wake-up call: stroke, diabetes, cancer, heart disease. I was 49, pre-diabetic, and sitting on a ticking time bomb. That was my moment.

So, I jumped into Keto. But man, I made it complicated.

I bought all the Keto "must-haves"—fancy shakes, ketone enhancers, MCT oils, protein bars, fat bombs, collagen powder… I was exhausted and broke. That's when I found Dr. Ken Berry on YouTube. His video ("3 First Steps to Going Keto – Credit Card NOT Required") changed everything.

You don't need fancy products. You don't need a meal plan. You just need to cut sugar and eat real food.

Here's what I did:

- Ate fatty meats (with the skin!)

- Cooked with real butter and olive oil

- Ate leafy green veggies

- Snacked on cheese, nuts (in moderation), pork rinds, and celery

- Drank lots of water—a gallon a day
- Ditched sugar completely (yep, even the "just one bite" kind)

I stopped weighing myself. I measured progress in my clothes. From size 18 to a size 5/6. I haven't worn that since middle school.

It's not about counting calories—it's about cutting sugar and letting your body heal.

Chapter 5: The Keto Experiment

Okay, your turn.

You've read this far, which means something deep inside you is DONE. Let's do something with that.

Step 1: Health Inventory

- Use an online health assessment (like [Healthy Life HRA](#))

- Talk to family about their health history

- Get bloodwork done. Be honest with your doctor about considering Keto

- Check in on your emotional and mental state

Step 2: Mindset

- **WHY** are you here? Be honest. Be raw. Yes, you're probably overweight. That's okay—we've all been there.

- **WHY** do you want to change? List it: health, marriage, confidence, peace.

- **HOW** did you get here? What behaviors, traumas, or beliefs caused this weight?

- **GET MAD**. Not at people. Not at your spouse or kids. But at what your weight has stolen from your life. That anger can push you into motion.

- **NOW RESOLVE TO CHANGE**. Food doesn't control you. YOU control you.

Step 3: Purge the Pantry

Get rid of the sugar, the chips, the crackers. Out of sight, out of reach.

Step 4: Plan for Eating Out

Don't wait until you're at the table to decide. Make a plan. No bun. No fries. Water, not soda. And order FIRST.

Step 5: Grace Over Guilt

If you mess up, don't quit. Don't wait for Monday. Just get back on track at your next meal. One choice doesn't erase your progress.

Step 6: Give It 3 Months

Be strict. Let your body adapt. It gets easier. I promise.

Step 7: Stop Weighing

Use clothes or a tape measure. A 5-pound loss might be
2 pant sizes. Trust the process.

Step 8: Eat Like This

- Fats: Avocado, olive oil, butter, coconut oil

- Proteins: Fatty cuts of meat, eggs, bacon, tuna, chicken

- Veggies: Greens, cauliflower, zucchini

- Snacks: Nuts (a handful!), cheese, celery with cream cheese, buffalo chicken dip

- Water: One gallon a day. Seriously.

Step 9: Ask Yourself Again—WHY?

Why are you doing this? Why now? Why YOU? (The
answer: Because you deserve it.)

Step 10: START.

Give it three months. No gimmicks. No starting Monday.
Just GO.

Chapter 6: Wait—What Can I Eat Again?!

So by now you might be thinking:
 "Okay, I'm ready to do this. But… what can I actually eat??"

Great question. Let's break it down, simple and straight.

What You CAN Eat on a Ketogenic Diet:

■ **1. Healthy Fats** – the good stuff.
 This is your main source of energy now. About 75–80% of your diet will come from fat. Don't panic—that's the point!

- **Real butter (yes, with a guilt-free smile)**

- **MCT oil**

- **Coconut oil**

- **Avocado oil**

- **Olive oil**

■ **2. Non-Starchy Vegetables** – your new carb crew.
 These are your only real carb sources. Stick with green, leafy veggies and cruciferous veggies.

- **Salad greens, spinach, kale**

- **Cucumber, celery, zucchini**

- **Broccoli, cauliflower, cabbage**
  These should be about 10–20% of your diet.

■ **3. Protein** – YES, meat lovers rejoice!
 Meat is back on the menu. Don't fear fat on meat—embrace it.

- **Eggs (nature's perfect food)**

- **Beef, pork, poultry**

- **Fish and shellfish**

- **Organ meats (yes, liver is a powerhouse)**

- **Full-fat dairy (not skim!)**

- **Bone broth (great for your gut and joints)**

■ **4. Beverages** – keep it clean.

- **Water (LOTS of it!)**

- **Unsweetened tea**

- Black coffee (or "bulletproof" with butter or MCT oil)

- Bone broth

■ **5. Extras – flavor without guilt.**

- **Herbs and spices**

- **Vinegar**

- **Hot sauce (check for added sugar!)**

- **Mustard (unsweetened)**

- **Stevia or monk fruit (sparingly)**

Be Cautious With These – Eat in Moderation:

▲ Cream cheese, sour cream, heavy cream
▲ Full-fat cheeses
▲ Canned coconut milk

These aren't "bad," but they're easy to overdo—especially if you're still learning how to listen to your hunger cues.

▲ Starchy veggies like:

- Carrots
- Sweet or regular potatoes
- Artichokes
- Beans and legumes (black beans, lima beans, etc.)

▲ Nuts and seeds:

- Almonds, cashews, walnuts

- Sunflower seeds, pumpkin seeds
  They're calorie-dense and easy to snack on mindlessly. Measure them if you're including them.

What to AVOID COMPLETELY:

🚫 Sugar and Sweeteners
That includes:

- White sugar
- Brown sugar
- Honey
- Maple syrup
- Agave
- Any "syrup"

🚫 Grains and Grain Products
Say goodbye to:

- Rice
- Oats
- Corn
- Tortillas
- Bread
- Pasta
- Grits

🚫 Processed Junk

- Chips
- Cereal
- Snack bars
- Pretzels
- Crackers

🚫 Sugary Drinks and Alcohol

- Soda
- Sweetened tea
- Juice
- Most alcohols (especially beer and sweet liquors)
  Even "sugar-free" products can be sneaky with artificial sweeteners that mess with your insulin.

The Simple Formula:

**Eat real fat-rich foods, green vegetables,
and drink plenty of water.**

That's it. It's not rocket science. You don't need a PhD in
nutrition. You need a plate with fat, protein, greens, and
a tall glass of water. Repeat daily.

Easy peasy, right? You're not starving. You're eating
real, satisfying food. No need to count calories or chase
macros unless you want to. Just stay away from sugar,
grains, and junk.

Sample Menu – One Day on Keto

🔍 **Breakfast:**
Bacon and eggs (over-easy, cooked in butter)

- **Black coffee or bulletproof coffee**

- **Water**

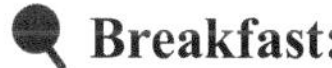**Lunch:**
Mixed greens salad

- **Grilled chicken breast**
- **Boiled egg**
- **Olive oil and vinegar dressing**

Dinner:
Grilled salmon fillet

- Steamed broccoli and zucchini
- Butter drizzle, salt, and pepper

Snack (if needed):
Lettuce wrap with ham, tomato, and sugar-free mayo
(Or celery sticks with cream cheese)

Now tell me doesn't that sound good!

Chapter 7: This Isn't a Diet—It's FREEDOM

I've said it before, but it's worth repeating:

Keto is NOT a diet.
 It's a lifestyle—one where you take your power back.

You're not counting points. You're not starving. You're not forcing yourself to eat cardboard-tasting "health" food. You're not going to bed hungry or waking up bloated.

You are eating real food. You are healing your body from the inside out. You are watching the weight fall off—not from magic, but from consistency and intention.

And the best part?
 You'll feel the difference long before you see it.

⚡ **More energy**
 ⚡ **Less brain fog**
 ⚡ **Better sleep**
 ⚡ **Less joint pain**
 ⚡ **Fewer mood swings**
 ⚡ **More confidence**

You are teaching your body how to thrive without sugar.
And once it learns—there's no going back.

Listen—food isn't the enemy. It's fuel.
 You're not punishing yourself by doing Keto. You're
empowering yourself.

So don't get lost in the "rules." Keep it simple.

Eat fat.
Eat protein.
Eat greens.
Drink water.
Repeat.

This isn't restriction—it's FREEDOM.
 Freedom from sugar crashes.
 Freedom from cravings.
 Freedom from emotional eating.
 Freedom from hating what you see in the mirror.

Chapter 8: Exercise – Just Move Your Body

Let me tell you what I did for exercise:
 I got off the couch. I turned off the TV. I put the phone down.
 I made time for ME.

At first? It wasn't easy. Life was already packed. I was working full-time, raising kids with busy sports schedules, and on top of that—I was a full-time college student. Sound familiar?

I had to create a plan that worked *for my life*, not some fantasy schedule. And guess what? So will you.

Where Can You Make Time?

Two miles from my house, there's a track I passed every day on my way home from work. There was also a YMCA nearby. The resources were there—I just had to figure out how to fit them into my day.

Here's what I did:
 I sat down and looked at my schedule. I asked myself:

- Where am I being productive (work, school, driving)?

- Where am I just sitting, doing nothing productive?

Even if I was sitting in the bleachers at a game or in my car waiting at practice, I realized—I could use that time. Instead of scrolling social media, I started walking around the school track, the parking lot, or driving over to the gym.

Sometimes, practice would end early, and I'd only get in ten minutes of movement. But that's ten more minutes of progress than I had before.

What My Routine Looked Like

Here's a rough outline of how I made it work:

1. Get off work

2. Hit the gym

3. Pick the kids up from practice
   Go home, do housework, cook dinner
   Eat

4. Let my food settle while I worked on college coursework

5. Then head out again—either to the track two miles away or run in circles in my own backyard for 30–45 minutes

Yep, I said it: running literal circles in the backyard. You do what you have to do!

Your Plan = Your Results

Now, I can't tell you what workout program will work best for *you*, because I don't know your goals. Want to lose fat? Build muscle? Improve stamina? Tone up?

Generally, what works best (based on everything I've read and tried) is:

■ **HIIT (High-Intensity Interval Training)**
■ **Cardio for 30 minutes, 3–4 times a week**
■ **Weight training for strength and body composition**

You know your body and what results you want. Explore sites like:

- Bodybuilding.com – workouts, meal plans, and goal-based training

- Beachbody.com – online programs with support

- YouTube – a treasure chest of free workouts, no matter your level

I personally downloaded the Bodybuilding.com app, BodySpace (it's free!), which helped me stay on track. It has workouts, support, and videos that show you exactly how to do each exercise properly.

I also used apps like Goals – Fitness Tracker to monitor my progress.

Before You Start—Talk to Your Doctor

Seriously—always check with your healthcare provider before starting any new fitness or nutrition plan. Every body is different, and there's no one-size-fits-all program.

That said, Bodybuilding.com and other platforms have tools for *everyone*: beginners, people over 40, fat-loss goals, toning, strength-building, you name it. You can choose your trainer, your focus, and your pace.

Bottom Line: Just Start

I get it—starting is the hardest part. But once I got going, it became easier.

Here's how you get started:

1. Pick a plan. (Find something that works for *your* life.)
 2. Set goals. (Fat loss? Strength? Energy?)
 3. Start. (Even if it's just 10 minutes.)
 4. Be consistent. (Consistency over perfection.)
 5. Don't quit. (Even if you stumble, don't stop.)

NEVER GIVE UP on your goals or your plan. Your health is worth it. YOU are worth it.

Chapter 9: Intermittent Fasting – What is THAT?

People have been fasting since before the birth of Christ. If you've ever read the Bible or heard the stories, you know that fasting was often a gateway to revelation, strength, and wisdom. It was also a way to practice self-control—which, let's be honest, is something a lot of us struggle with. Biblically speaking, a lack of self-control is often at the root of choices that harm our health and well-being.

Whether you're spiritual or not, there's no denying the emotional and cognitive benefits tied to Intermittent Fasting. And when you combine Intermittent Fasting with Keto, the results can be amazing—for your mind, your body, and your soul.

How Does Intermittent Fasting Work?

According to the American Heart Association (heart.org), research shows that intermittent fasting is linked to lower heart failure rates and even longer lifespans.

Dr. Satchidananda Panda, featured in an article by AHA News, explains that intermittent fasting helps keep the mitochondria in your heart healthy by reducing certain proteins related to ATP production. Translation? It lowers oxidative stress and gives your body time to repair itself. That's huge!

Benefits of Intermittent Fasting (IF)

One study published on the National Institutes of Health website outlines some serious perks of time-restricted eating. These include:

- Improved cardiovascular health

- Lower blood pressure

- Potential treatment and prevention for Type 2 Diabetes

> **Study Source:** *Malinowski B, Zalewska K, Węsierska A, Sokołowska MM, Socha M, Liczner G, Pawlak-Osińska K, Wiciński M. Intermittent Fasting in Cardiovascular Disorders-An Overview. Nutrients. 2019 Mar 20;11(3):673. doi: 10.3390/nu11030673. PMID: 30897855; PMCID: PMC6471315. https://pmc.ncbi.nlm.nih.gov/articles/PMC6471315/*

Intermittent fasting also boosts your body's ability to produce ketones—which you know from earlier chapters are powerhouses for fat burning and brain function.

In fact, animal studies suggest that intermittent fasting might reduce cognitive decline, and researchers are even exploring it as a possible treatment for Alzheimer's and dementia.

> Alzheimer's research: *Cummings, J. L., Isaacson, R. S., Mills, R., Williams, H., Chiulli, A., Perdomo, C. A., ... Fillit, H. (2021). Alzheimer's disease: Targeting risk reduction and early detection of cognitive decline with noninvasive approaches. Alzheimer's & Dementia: Translational Research & Clinical Interventions, 7(1), e12168. https://doi.org/10.1002/trc2.12168*

One fascinating study I came across found that fasting can stimulate the body's natural growth hormone (HGH) production, which helps maintain homeostasis—your body's internal balance. That's big for energy, muscle retention, fat burning, and more.

> **Growth hormone and fasting:** *Ho KY, Veldhuis JD, Johnson ML, Furlanetto R, Evans WS, Alberti KG, Thorner MO. Fasting enhances growth hormone secretion and amplifies the complex rhythms of growth hormone secretion in man. J Clin Invest. 1988 Apr;81(4):968-75. doi: 10.1172/JCI113450. PMID: 3127426; PMCID: PMC329619. https://pmc.ncbi.nlm.nih.gov/articles/PMC 329619/*

So, What *Is* Intermittent Fasting?

In simple terms, Intermittent Fasting (IF) is a pattern of eating and not eating. It's not about *what* you eat—it's about *when* you eat.

Two of the most popular methods are:

- **16:8 Fast (also called the Leangains Protocol): Fast for 16 hours, eat during an 8-hour window. You can fit 1 to 3 meals in that eating window.**

- **18:6 Fast: Fast for 18 hours, eat during a 6-hour window. Same concept, just a bit more fasting.**

In an article from PopSugar, Dr. Jason Fung (a nephrologist and author of *The Complete Guide to Fasting*) explains how intermittent fasting boosts HGH and lowers insulin levels—which means more fat burning, especially around the belly.

> **PopSugar article:** *Sandler, M. (2019, January 14). What is 18:6 intermittent fasting? PopSugar.*
> *https://www.popsugar.com/fitness/What-18 6-Intermittent-Fasting-45446501*

Institude for Functional Medicine:
Institute for Functional Medicine. (n.d.).
Intermittent fasting and heart health
[Audio podcast]. IFM.
https://www.ifm.org/podcast/intermittent-fasting-and-heart-health

---

Why Did *I* Start Fasting?

I started intermittent fasting for the cognitive boost and HGH benefits. As a middle-aged woman, I wanted to do something that would support my health through this next phase of life—and help me *feel* good and function at my best.

I've had family members and friends say I look younger, and honestly, I *feel* younger. I have more energy, mental clarity, and I'm not constantly crashing throughout the day.

Yes, the weight loss helped. But I believe intermittent fasting played a huge role in restoring my confidence, focus, and peace of mind.

Fasting + Keto = Real Results

Both Keto and IF encourage the body to produce
ketones, which help burn fat—especially stubborn belly
fat. They also support:

- Heart health

- Blood sugar control

- Reduced anxiety and brain fog

Before Keto and IF, my body was all over the place. I
was tired, cranky, bloated, and sick of feeling out of
control. I didn't like how I looked, how I felt, or how I
was showing up in life.

But within six months of committing to Keto and
Intermittent Fasting, I lowered my:

- Blood pressure

- Cholesterol

- Glucose levels

And I gained my mental clarity, confidence, and sanity
back.

Take Back Control

Here's the deal: YOU DO YOU.
 This is your life, your health, your journey.

You have to decide what's right for you and why you're doing it. I can't do that part for you. But what I *can* say is this: I'm proud of how far I've come. I feel great, I look better, and I'm finally in control again.

> *Food no longer controls me—I control it.*
> *I decide when, where, and what I eat.*

There was a time when food ruled my life. I'd go to a party and binge "just because it was a special occasion." I'd buy a whole box of Little Debbie Nutty Bars and hide the wrappers out of shame. I hated what I saw in the mirror and blamed the food… but really, it was about control.

Now? I'm in charge.

Are you ready to take back that control, too?

Chapter 10: Before and After – Take Plenty of Pictures

Let me tell you something: one of the most powerful things I ever did on this journey was take photos—lots of them.

When I look at my "after" pictures now, I sometimes still can't believe it's me. I made sure to use similar facial angles so the difference would be clear—and wow, the transformation is undeniable. Not just in my body, but in my *eyes*. You know how people say you can tell a lot from someone's eyes? I believe that now. There's a new light in mine. Can you see it? That energy, confidence, and joy? It's real. And it came from doing the work, sticking with it, and giving myself the chance to change.

If you're starting Keto and Intermittent Fasting, prepare to witness some pretty amazing changes—especially in your face and abdomen. Those are usually the first areas to show visible progress. And beyond what you see, you'll start *feeling* the difference: more energy, less bloat, clearer skin, better sleep, and a stronger mindset.

Take That First Photo

I know it can feel awkward or even painful to take those "before" pictures—but do it anyway. Trust me, you'll be glad you did.

Here's how to get started:

- Men: Take photos in shorts, no shirt.

- Women: Try running shorts and a sports bra, or a bikini.

- Take three angles: front, side, and back.

- Keep them private: Store the photos somewhere only *you* can see, unless you decide to share your progress later.

Then—do it again. Every month. Preferably in the same outfit, same poses, same lighting. That way, the changes stand out.

It Was Never About the Scale

For me, it wasn't about the number on the scale. It was about how I *felt*—and let's be honest, I felt fat. I measured success by my jeans size, how my clothes fit, and how I moved through my day. Honestly? I threw the scale out.

Instead, I went shopping for jeans in a smaller size—even before I could fit in them. Those jeans became my motivation. I'd try them on each month just to see how close I was. And let me tell you—zipping them up for the first time? That feeling was better than seeing any number on a scale.

The Yarn Trick

Another method I loved was what I call the "yarn method." It's super simple, cheap, and powerful.

Here's what you do:

1. Take a piece of yarn and wrap it around your abdomen.

2. Cut it to the exact length it takes to go around.

3. Save it—maybe tape it to a piece of poster board and write the date on it.

4. Each month, repeat the process with a new piece of yarn.

5. After a few months, line them up side-by-side.

You'll be amazed at the difference. It's a visual, physical reminder of how far you've come—and that's the kind of motivation that hits different.

Celebrate Progress – Even the Small Stuff

This journey isn't about perfection—it's about progress. And sometimes, when you're deep in it, it's hard to notice just how much you're changing. That's why photos and yarn work so well. They give you proof. They remind you that your hard work is *working*, even when the mirror or the scale seems stubborn.

So take those pictures. Save those yarn loops. Celebrate those non-scale victories.

You're changing. You're growing. And soon, you'll be looking at your "after" photo thinking, *"Wow... that really is me."*

Chapter 11: What I Do... Plain and Simple

I'll be honest—I wanted to rush through this part. Just blaze right through it, wild and free, and get to the finish line. But then I realized, if I don't slow down and share the *actual things I do*, I'd be leaving you without the most important part: how to start.

So here it is. Plain and simple. No fluff. No gimmicks. Just what works for me.

Mornings Start with Coffee... and Oil

I drink a *lot* of coffee. Like, probably more than I should admit. But I don't just drink it—I boost it. I add MCT oil (that's medium-chain triglycerides), which comes from coconuts and has been shown in some studies to help with weight loss and metabolic health.

I pour it straight into my coffee, especially when I'm breaking a fast. Yes, it's a little oily at first, but it's not gross. It's got this smooth, dry oil feel that I actually kind of like now. Think of dry oil like something you'd put on your skin—it absorbs quickly and doesn't leave you feeling greasy.

This combo is what most people call "Bulletproof Coffee," originally made popular by Dave Asprey (you can look him up if you want to go down that rabbit hole). Supposedly, it kickstarts your brain and metabolism first thing in the morning. All I know is: it helps me stay focused and feel sharp—so I drink it. Especially when I'm doing a 16:8 or 18:6 fasting schedule. It gets me through to my first meal without a problem.

So, What Do I Actually Eat?

People always ask, "What does a typical meal look like for you?"

Here's the lowdown:

- I love canned chicken or tuna. I mix it with Duke's mayo (because it has no sugar and tastes bomb), and eat it on a bed of lettuce with cucumbers, broccoli, and sugar-free ranch—or homemade dressing if I'm feeling fancy.

- For breakfast, I'm all about steak and eggs. Cooked in real butter. Not grass-fed. Just butter. The good kind. If a T-bone's in the budget, that's what I'm eating.

- For the family, I make crustless pizza or pizza casseroles—meat, cheese, low-sugar marinara, veggies. No bread. No crust. All the good stuff.

- I also make stuffed zucchini using the same toppings as my pizza casserole. Add some buffalo chicken dip on the side with pork rinds, celery, or cucumbers—chef's kiss.

When I need ideas, I just type "Keto recipes" into Google and pick something easy I think the family won't turn their noses up at.

Nuts, Seeds, and Oils—My Pantry Staples

- I use flaxseed sprinkled on my food.

- I snack on walnuts, macadamias, pecans, and Brazil nuts—but not too many. Nuts are healthy, but they still have carbs. I pre-measure two small servings in little bowls or snack bags and call it a day.

I cook everything in avocado oil, olive oil, coconut oil, or real butter. I also load up on herbs and spices to keep things interesting.

And when it comes to veggies, my rule is:
"Lean is green."
So I stick to green vegetables—broccoli, lettuce, cabbage, Brussels sprouts, spinach, asparagus, green onions, peppers… you get the idea.

Fat Bombs? Oh Yeah.

When I need a snack or a treat, I whip up some coconut oil fat bombs. A fat bomb is exactly what it sounds like—a little snack made mostly of healthy fat. Coconut oil is solid at room temperature below 78 degrees, so these babies live in the fridge.

And yes—I'll share some recipes. Calm down, y'all. I got you.

Do I Follow a Plan?

Honestly? Not really.

That's the beauty of Keto. I don't need a strict "plan." I just keep my house stocked with:

- Healthy fats (avocados, cheese, coconut oil, MCT oil, olive oil, pork rinds, nuts)

- Healthy proteins

- Green veggies

If it's not one of those things... I don't eat it. That simple.

Wait... What About Macros?

Listen—I don't track macros. I barely know what they are. Unless we're talking macaroni and cheese, in which case... I still don't want to know.

This isn't that kind of book. I'm not a scientist. I'm not a nutritionist. I'm just a girl who found something that worked and felt too good not to share.

I'm not claiming to be the queen of Keto or the guru of Fasting. I'm just the master of me.

And that's what I want for you—to become the master of YOU.

That's why we started this whole thing with a lifestyle inventory. That's why I had you dig into your family health history. And most importantly, that's why we focused on mindset from the **beginning.**

**Remember Chapter 2?
 Mindset is EVERYTHING.**

You Thought You Were Ready... But Were You?

I knew if I hit you with too much mindset stuff early on, you'd be like, "Boring! Tell me about bacon!" ●

But here's the truth: you probably thought you were ready to jump in headfirst. And then you kept reading... and you weren't so sure anymore. Then you saw my before-and-after photos, and that lit a little fire under you. Am I right?

It's okay. That's all part of the process.

Coming Up Next...

In the next chapter, I'm diving into practical strategies for *actually changing your mindset*. Tools, links, resources—stuff you can use every day to keep the fire going long after the "honeymoon phase" wears off.

Because as exciting as that first week of results is... you'll need something deeper to keep going.

And yes—as I'm writing this—I still haven't picked a title for this book. I'm waiting until this journey fully unfolds. Because that's how I roll.

Ready to shift your mindset for good?

Good. Let's go.

Chapter 12: MOTIVATIONAL RESOURCES

Well... here we go.

Let me just say this upfront—**motivation looks different for everyone**. For me, the biggest push came from my children. I wanted to *be there*—not just physically present, but healthy, active, and engaged as they grew up. I wanted to be around long enough to meet my grandkids, to spoil them rotten, and to have the kind of relationship with them that my kids never got to have with their grandparents.

That still gets me emotional.
 Because honestly? One of the biggest injustices in life is a child growing up without the love of good, warm, devoted grandparents. I never wanted that cycle to repeat.

And then there was me.
 My **health**, my **energy**, my **body**, my **mind**—they were all spiraling. I could feel it in my career, in my schoolwork, in how I talked to people... even in how I talked to *myself*. I was mentally and physically tired. And not just "I need a nap" tired. I mean the kind of soul-exhausted that makes you feel like you're living on autopilot.

That was the wake-up call.
 And right around that time, I was required to take a *lifestyle* class. Talk about divine timing. That class

opened the door to something bigger—a different way to think, eat, move, and live. That's when I realized: if I didn't change things, **nothing was going to change**.

Side note: If you want to take a free class on lifestyle stuff, there are tons online. Check out Skillshare.com if you need a place to start. Not sponsored, just helpful. In fact, I've even thought about creating my own course someday.

Anyway, back to motivation.

So... What Motivates YOU?

I've told you what got me fired up. Now it's your turn.

Maybe it's your health.
 Maybe it's your clothes not fitting.
 Maybe it's a dream vacation you want to feel confident taking.
 Maybe it's wanting to feel sexy for your spouse—or just for yourself.
 Maybe you want to feel alive again.

Whatever it is, OWN IT.
 Don't let anyone else define it for you. Not your partner, not your mom, not your best friend. **Only you** know what truly drives you.

When you figure it out, let it *fuel your fire*. Billy Alsbrooks calls it "lighter fluid"—that one thing that sets everything ablaze and gets you *moving*. Hold on to that. Write it down. Say it out loud. Repeat it when you want to quit.

And if you *don't* know what motivates you yet? That's okay too.

Start exploring. Watch motivational videos. Read self-help books. Listen to podcasts. I promise—something will eventually hit you like lightning. When it does, grab it and don't let go.

So... Who Helped Me Get Started?

When I first started Keto, I had *no clue* what I was doing.

Where did I go?
 You guessed it—**YouTube**.

I typed in "Keto," and up popped **Dr. Ken Berry**. He's the author of *Lies My Doctor Told Me*, and his videos were the *perfect* intro for someone like me who didn't know a carb from a ketone.

Start with his video "Three Steps to Going on Keto" and another one called "What is Keto?"—they're short, simple, and packed with exactly what you need to get going.
 Here's a link if you want to check him out:

👉 [Dr. Ken Berry's YouTube Channel:](https://youtu.be/xwKmVjSXTDk)
https://youtu.be/xwKmVjSXTDk

He made Keto sound doable. Budget-friendly. No special shakes or pills. That was all I needed to hear.

Work Challenge + Instant Results = Fire Lit

Another HUGE motivator was the **"Weigh Down Challenge"** at work.

It started in January. I told myself I was going to **win**—and I did. In the first *month*, I lost 15 pounds. Within 4-5 months, I dropped 60. The fat just started melting off. I couldn't believe how fast it happened. I could see it in my waist, my face, my energy, my confidence.

That kind of success becomes its own motivation. You don't want to stop once you feel that kind of momentum.

But Then... The Plateau

After about a year, my weight loss hit a wall. Plateau city.

I got discouraged. A little voice crept in: "Maybe this is it. Maybe you've gone as far as you can go."

Nope. Not today, Satan.

I started listening to **motivational speakers**. And guess where I found them?
 Yep—**YouTube**, again.

Let me give you some names:

- **Billy Alsbrooks** (his energy is on another level)

- **Dwayne "The Rock" Johnson** (obviously)

- **Inky Johnson** (you'll cry in the best way)

- **Matthew McConaughey** (deep stuff)

- **Denzel Washington** (wisdom for days)

- **Andy Frisella** – His *RealAF* podcast got me back in the zone

Most of their stuff is on Spotify, too. Just start playing around. Someone's words will hit your heart.

Even My Music Changed

I even switched up my music when I started running.

I went from chill vibes to **full-on beast mode**:
 Seether. Disturbed. Breaking Benjamin. Godsmack.

Killswitch Engage. Korn. Five Finger Death Punch. I needed *fire*. I needed something that made me want to punch the air and scream, "LET'S GO!"

If that's not your style, no worries. Find music that gets *you* moving.

Books, Tools, and Tips

If reading's more your thing, check out books by **Billy Alsbrooks** and **Andy Frisella**. Or just search "motivational books" on Amazon. Whatever lights your fire—go for it.

Here are a few more ideas to stay motivated:

- **Accountability partner** – Grab a friend or coworker and do this together. Even better if they're just as hyped as you are.

- **Journal** – Track your wins, your struggles, your "aha" moments. It helps you spot what's working and what's not.

- **Take pictures** – I'm saying this AGAIN because it's THAT important. Photos don't lie. They show your growth when the scale doesn't.

- **Measure, don't weigh** – Forget the scale. Use clothes, measuring tape, even yarn if you have to. Focus on size, strength, and how you *feel.*

- 🧠 **Set goals** – Write them down. Big ones, small ones. Dream goals. Real goals. Let your goals become your *reality*.

Last Thing...

I can't tell you exactly what's going to spark that change inside of you.
 But I *can* tell you this:

Once you find it—everything changes.

You'll stop making excuses.
 You'll stop waiting for "Monday."
 You'll stop wondering if it's worth it.
 And you'll start becoming the YOU that's been buried under years of stress, habits, pain, fear, and doubt.

Your job now is to figure out what lights you up—and then pour gasoline on it.

Because once that fire gets going?
 Ain't nothing stopping you.

Let's go.

Chapter 13
Somebody Say RECIPE?

Ohhhh yes, I did promise you some recipes! And honey, when I say these got me through the cravings and kept me from diving face-first into a pizza, I mean it. These are my go-to "keep-me-sane" snacks and meals—super simple, super satisfying, and absolutely packed with fat (so if you're not doing Keto, consider yourself warned). But for my fellow Keto warriors? Let's eat!

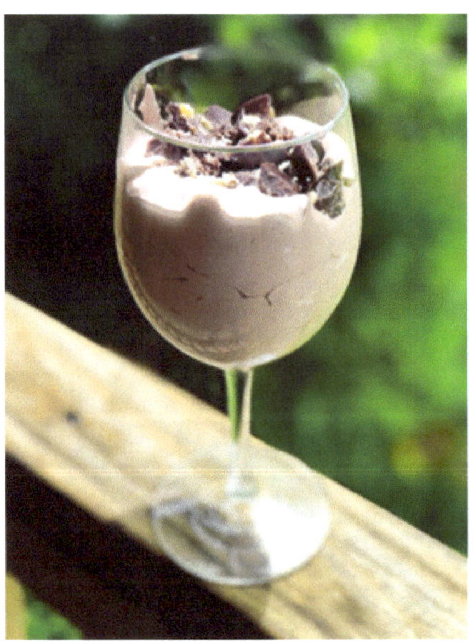

◆ *Keto Chocolate Frosty*

This one hits every single sweet tooth craving without sending your insulin on a rollercoaster ride. It's like a Wendy's Frosty but with none of the guilt.

Ingredients

- 1½ cups heavy whipping cream

- 3 tablespoons Swerve Confectioners (or your fave powdered keto sweetener)

- Pinch of kosher salt
- 2 tablespoons unsweetened cocoa powder
- 1 teaspoon vanilla extract (optional)

Topping

- Crushed Chocolate Fat Bomb (see next recipe), sugar-free chocolate chips, or chopped nuts

Directions
1. Whisk all ingredients in a large bowl until stiff peaks form. (You can use a hand mixer for speed.)

2. Scoop into a zip-top freezer bag and freeze until semi-firm—don't go full ice cream here!

3. Snip the corner of the bag and squeeze into a dessert dish like frosting.

4. Add toppings and enjoy like the keto royalty you are.

◆ *Chocolate Fat Bombs*

These are lifesavers. I keep a stash in my freezer at all times.

Ingredients

- 2 heaping tablespoons solid coconut oil
- 2 heaping tablespoons cocoa powder
- 2 tablespoons Swerve confectioners (or 5 packets Stevia)

Optional Add-Ins

- Nuts (walnuts, pecans, black walnuts… get wild)

Directions

1. Add all ingredients to a microwave-safe bowl.
2. Microwave for about 30–35 seconds.
3. Whisk until smooth.
4. Pour into silicone molds.
5. Freeze until solid (5–10 minutes). Done and delicious!

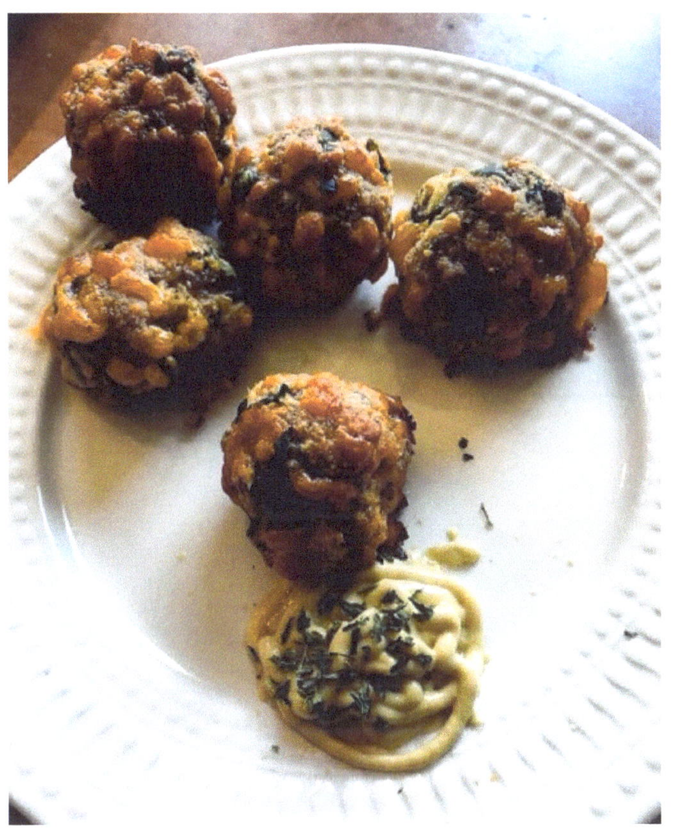

Keto Sausage Balls (Party Favorite)

These are a hit at every gathering. Trust me—people won't even know they're keto.

Ingredients

- 1 pound spicy ground pork sausage
- ½ (8 oz) block cream cheese, room temp
- ½ cup shredded extra sharp cheddar

- ½ cup grated Parmesan
- 1 tablespoon Dijon mustard
- 1 teaspoon garlic powder
- 1 teaspoon black pepper

Directions

1. Preheat oven to 375°F.
2. Mix all ingredients by hand in a large bowl.
3. Form into golf ball-sized pieces and place on a nonstick baking sheet.
4. Bake for 30–35 minutes or until golden brown.
5. Let cool slightly and serve with extra Dijon if you like dipping!

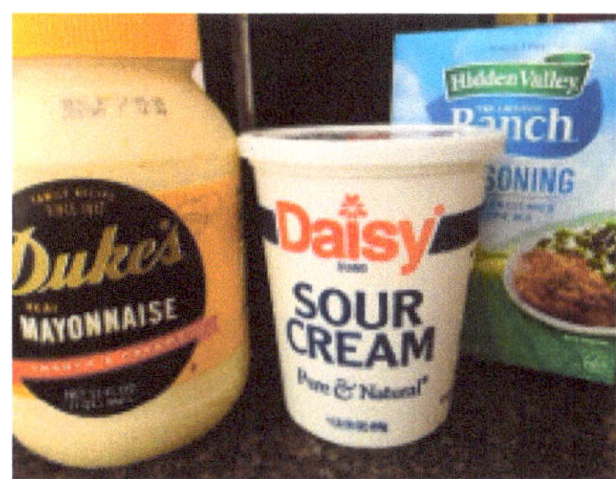 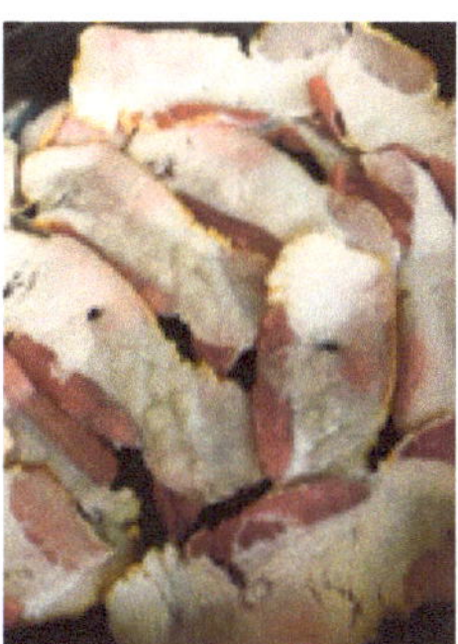

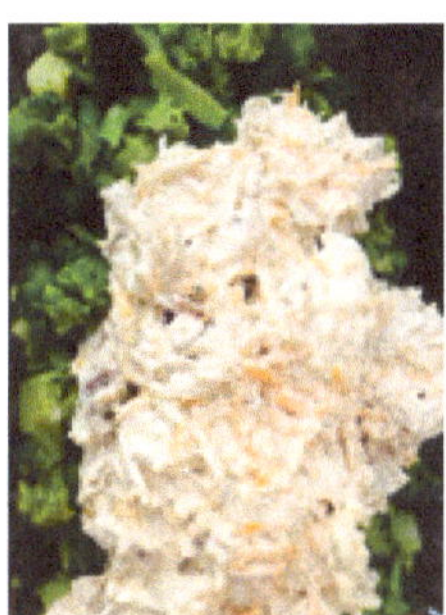 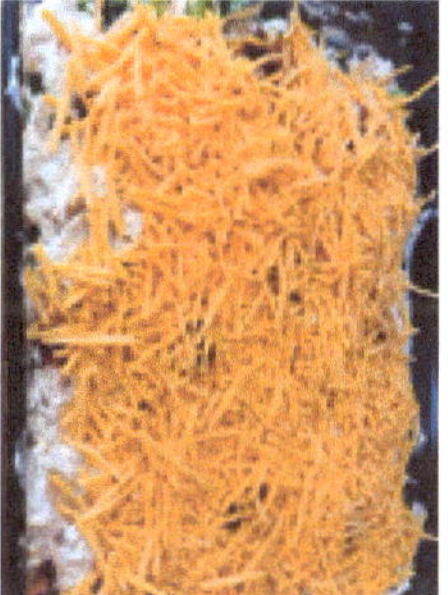

 *Chicken, Broccoli & Cheese Bake*

Total comfort food vibes without the carb coma.

Ingredients

- ½ cup mayonnaise

- ½ cup sour cream

- 1 packet ranch seasoning

- 10 oz chopped fresh broccoli (don't use frozen, it gets soggy)

- 1½ cups shredded sharp cheddar cheese

- 1¼ cups shredded cooked chicken

- ½ cup cooked bacon, crumbled

Topping

- 1 cup extra shredded cheddar

Directions

1. Preheat oven to 400°F.
2. Place broccoli at the bottom of a baking dish.
3. Mix mayo, sour cream, ranch mix, bacon, cheddar, and chicken.
4. Spread mixture over the broccoli and top with the extra cheese.
5. Bake for 30–35 minutes. Gooey, melty, satisfying.

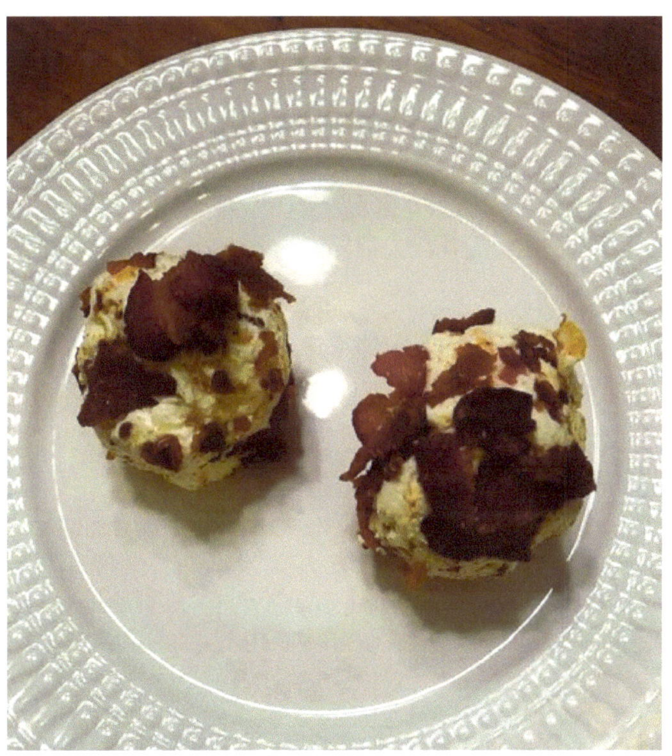

🌶 *Jalapeño Popper Fat Bombs*

If you love a little heat, you're going to be obsessed.

Ingredients

- 4 oz cream cheese, softened
- 1½ cups shredded sharp cheddar
- ½ cup jarred jalapeños, drained and chopped
- 6 slices crispy cooked bacon, chopped
- 1 tablespoon ranch seasoning
- 1 tablespoon garlic powder

Directions

1. Cook and crumble bacon.

2. Mix all ingredients (except bacon) and roll into bite-sized balls.

3. Roll each ball in bacon crumbles.

4. Serve fresh. Great for snacks or parties!

🍗 *Cheese Crisps*

No real recipe here—I wing it!
 Grab shredded extra sharp cheddar, mix in seasoning (ranch mix, chili powder, or garlic powder), and bake spoonfuls on parchment paper at 375°F until bubbly and golden. Let cool and crisp up. BOOM—keto chips!

🍕 *Crustless Pizza Casserole*

This one's a family favorite. No crust, no problem.

Ingredients

- Sugar-free marinara or pizza sauce

- Cooked meats: sausage, pepperoni, ham, ground beef

- Veggies: onions, olives, bell peppers
- Lots of shredded mozzarella cheese

Directions

1. Spread sauce in a baking dish.
2. Layer with meats and veggies.
3. Top with tons of cheese.
4. Bake at 400°F for about 20–25 minutes, until bubbly.

🌶 *Bacon-Wrapped Jalapeños*

Spicy, cheesy, bacon-wrapped goodness. Enough said.

Ingredients

- Fresh jalapeños, halved and seeded
- Cream cheese
- Shredded cheddar
- Garlic & onion powder
- Bacon strips

Directions

1. Mix cream cheese, cheddar, and seasoning.
2. Fill each jalapeño half with the mixture.
3. Wrap with bacon.
4. Bake at 400°F until bacon is browned and slightly crispy.

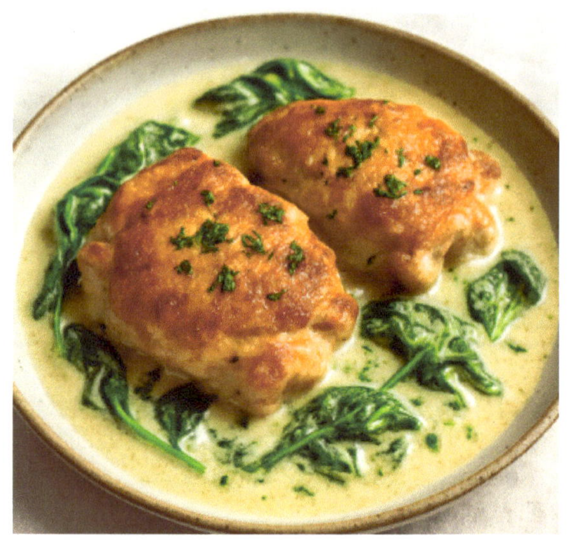

Creamy Garlic Parmesan Chicken (Keto)

🍳 **Ingredients:**

- 2 tbsp olive oil or avocado oil

- 4 boneless, skinless chicken thighs or breasts

- Salt and pepper to taste

- 3 cloves garlic, minced

- 1 cup heavy cream

- ½ cup grated Parmesan cheese

- 1 tsp Italian seasoning

- 1 cup spinach (optional, but great for nutrients and color)

- ¼ tsp crushed red pepper flakes (optional, for a little kick)
- 1 tbls. butter

Directions:

1. **Season the Chicken**: Sprinkle both sides of the chicken with salt and pepper.

2. **Sear the Chicken**:
   Heat the oil in a large skillet over medium heat.
   Sear the chicken for about 5-6 minutes per side, or until golden brown and cooked through.
   Remove chicken and set aside.

3. **Make the Cream Sauce**:
   In the same skillet, lower the heat and add garlic. Sauté for about 30 seconds until fragrant.
   Pour in the heavy cream, butter, and bring to a gentle simmer.
   Stir in Parmesan cheese, Italian seasoning, and red pepper flakes. Stir until melted and smooth.

4. **Add Spinach (optional)**:
   Stir in the spinach and cook until wilted (2–3 minutes).

5. **Combine and Serve**:
   Return the chicken to the pan and spoon sauce over the top. Let it simmer together for a couple of minutes.
   Serve hot, optionally over cauliflower rice or with roasted veggies.

This dish is rich in fats and protein while keeping carbs low—perfect for staying in ketosis. Using chicken thighs adds more flavor and fat, which is great for keto.

Berry Mascarpone Cloud Cups

Description:
 A creamy, whipped mascarpone base with vanilla and a hint of lemon zest, topped with fresh keto-friendly berries and a sugar-free berry glaze, served in individual dessert cups.

Ingredients (Serves 4):

Mascarpone Cream:

- 8 oz mascarpone cheese, softened

- 1/2 cup heavy whipping cream

- 2 tbsp powdered erythritol (or your preferred keto sweetener)

- 1/2 tsp vanilla extract
- 1/2 tsp lemon zest

Berry Topping:

- 1/2 cup raspberries

- 1/2 cup blackberries

- 1/4 cup blueberries

- 1 tbsp chia seeds (optional for thickening the glaze)

- 1 tbsp water

- 1 tbsp powdered erythritol

Optional Garnish:

- Fresh mint leaves

- Lemon zest curls

Directions:

1. **Make the Mascarpone Cream:**
    In a mixing bowl, whisk the mascarpone, heavy cream, sweetener, vanilla, and lemon zest together using a hand mixer until light, fluffy, and smooth (about 2-3 minutes). Chill while you make the topping.

2. **Prepare the Berry Glaze:**
    In a small saucepan, combine half the raspberries and blackberries with the water and erythritol over medium heat. Stir and mash the berries gently until they break down. Simmer for 5–7 minutes until thickened. Add chia seeds to help it gel (optional). Let it cool.

3. **Assemble the Cups:**
    Spoon the mascarpone cream into 4 small dessert glasses or ramekins. Top with a few fresh berries, then drizzle the berry glaze on top.

4. **Garnish and Serve:**
   Add a sprig of mint or a curl of lemon zest for garnish. Serve immediately or chill until ready to enjoy.

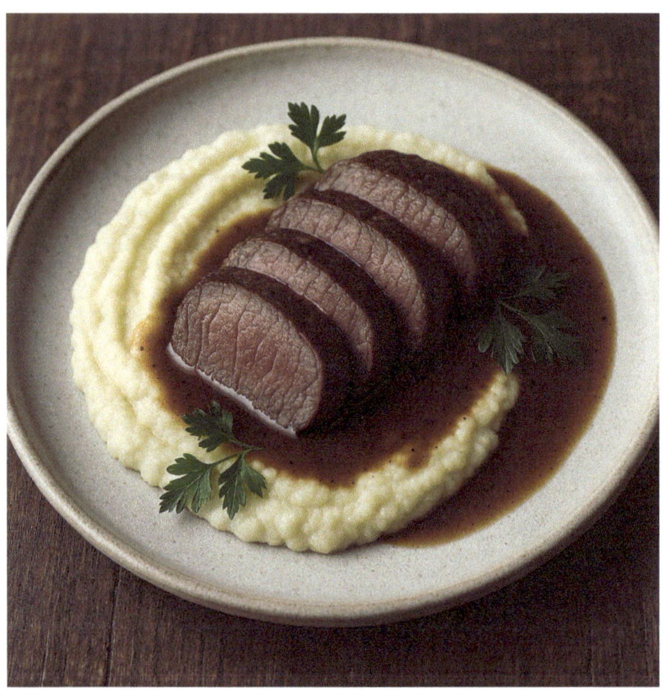

Garlic Herb Venison Medallions with Cauliflower Purée

Description:
Seared venison tenderloin medallions marinated in garlic, rosemary, and olive oil, served over a creamy cauliflower purée with a drizzle of herb-infused pan sauce.

Ingredients (Serves 2–3):

For the Venison:

- 1 lb venison tenderloin, sliced into 1-inch medallions
- 2 tbsp olive oil
- 2 cloves garlic, minced
- 1 tsp fresh rosemary, chopped
- 1 tsp fresh thyme, chopped
- Salt and pepper to taste

For the Cauliflower Purée:

- 1 small head of cauliflower, chopped
- 2 tbsp butter
- 2 tbsp heavy cream
- Salt and pepper to taste
- Optional: 1 tbsp grated Parmesan

Pan Sauce (optional):

- 1/4 cup beef broth
- 1 tbsp butter
- Splash of red wine vinegar or balsamic vinegar
- Fresh thyme sprig

Instructions:

1. **Marinate the Venison:**
    Combine olive oil, garlic, rosemary, thyme, salt, and pepper in a bowl. Toss venison medallions in the mixture and marinate for at least 30 minutes (or overnight for deeper flavor).

2. **Make the Cauliflower Purée:**
    Steam the cauliflower until tender (about 10 minutes). Blend in a food processor with butter, cream, salt, pepper, and optional Parmesan until smooth and creamy. Set aside, keep warm.

3. **Sear the Venison:**
    Heat a skillet over medium-high heat. Sear medallions for 2–3 minutes per side until browned and cooked to medium-rare or preferred doneness. Remove and let rest.

4. **Make the Pan Sauce (Optional):**
    In the same pan, add broth and vinegar, scraping browned bits. Simmer for 2–3 minutes, stir in butter and thyme. Reduce slightly and drizzle over the meat.

5. **Serve:**
    Spoon cauliflower purée onto plates, top with venison medallions, and drizzle with pan sauce. Garnish with extra herbs if desired.

Let's be real for a second—I don't measure much. I cook with my soul, not a spreadsheet. I experiment and adjust until I get it the way I like it. So don't stress if your version looks a little different. That's the beauty of Keto: it's flexible and forgiving.

I've started sharing more recipes on my blog—check them out when you need fresh ideas or just wanna see what I'm cookin' up next:
👉 Samara Hardee – Relentless Keto and IF : _http://samarahardee.blogspot.com_

So there you have it, my friend. These recipes helped me stay on track when temptation was knocking, and I hope they do the same for you. Keep it simple, make it tasty, and keep fighting forward. You got this!

Chapter 14

Final Word

Well friend, here we are—at the end of this book, but hopefully just the beginning of *your* transformation.

I've poured everything I know, everything I've tried, and everything that has worked for *me* into these pages. If even one sentence here helped you feel less alone or more equipped to take that next step in your Keto and Intermittent Fasting journey, then it's all been worth it.

I'm still learning, still growing, and still experimenting. I don't have it all figured out—but I've come far enough to know that *consistency beats perfection*, and your best tool is *not giving up*. If you want to stay connected, follow me on my blog:

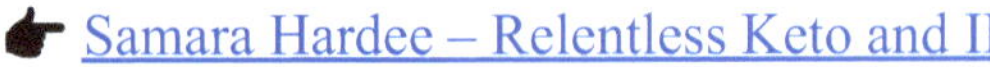 Samara Hardee – Relentless Keto and IF

I'm planning to launch a podcast soon—something real and relatable about healthy living, Keto, mindset, and more. My daily commute gives me plenty of time to think, reflect, and create. Once the podcast is up and running, I'll post the link on my blog so you won't miss a thing.

In the meantime, YouTube is an amazing resource. I highly recommend checking out Dr. Ken Berry and Dr. Eric Berg. They have completely different teaching styles, but both offer a ton of wisdom for living a low-carb, healthy lifestyle.

And yes—videos are coming too. I'd love to start making educational and inspirational YouTube content, so keep your eye on the blog for updates.

From the bottom of my heart, thank you for reading this book. Thank you for trusting me with part of your journey. This isn't just about weight loss—it's about reclaiming your life, your energy, your joy. And if I can do it, so can you.

I've also been thinking about giving back. While I haven't worked out all the details just yet, I'd like to donate a portion of the proceeds from this book to support domestic violence survivors. Once I choose the right organization, I'll share more on the blog.

This journey? It's yours. I'm just honored to walk alongside you for a little while.

Here's what I've learned:

- Health isn't just diet and exercise—it's *perspective*, it's *peace*, it's *purpose*.

- Your mental and emotional health matter just as much as the number on the scale.

- YOU matter.

- And you don't have to be perfect—just *persistent*.

Take time to unplug. Meditate. Dream. Listen to motivational podcasts. Read books that uplift your spirit. Fill your cup, because no one else can do that for you.

You are the captain of your own life. You get to steer the ship.

I'll leave you with this: **YOU do YOU.**
Because there is no one else in the world like you—and that, my friend, is your superpower.

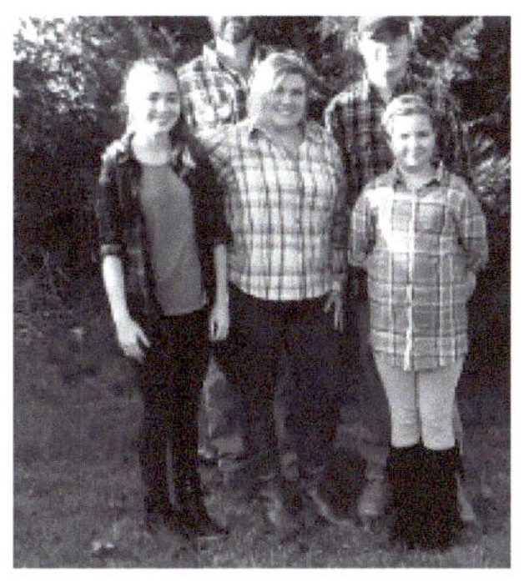 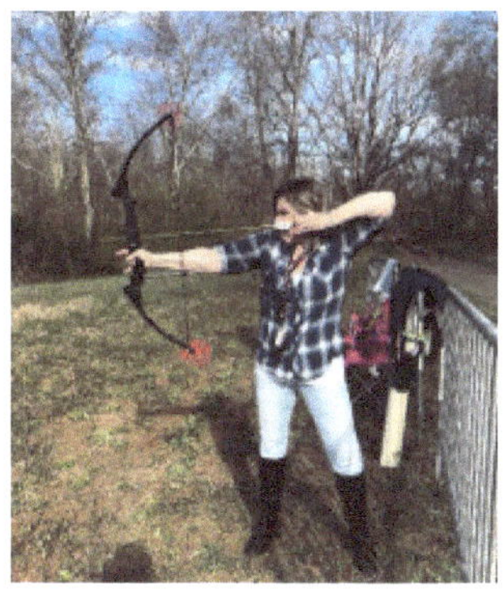

Progress pictures I had taken along the way….
When I realized I had a tiny little waist I was elated

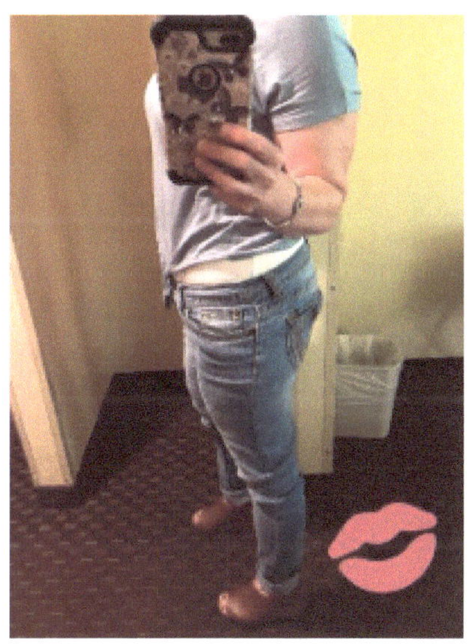

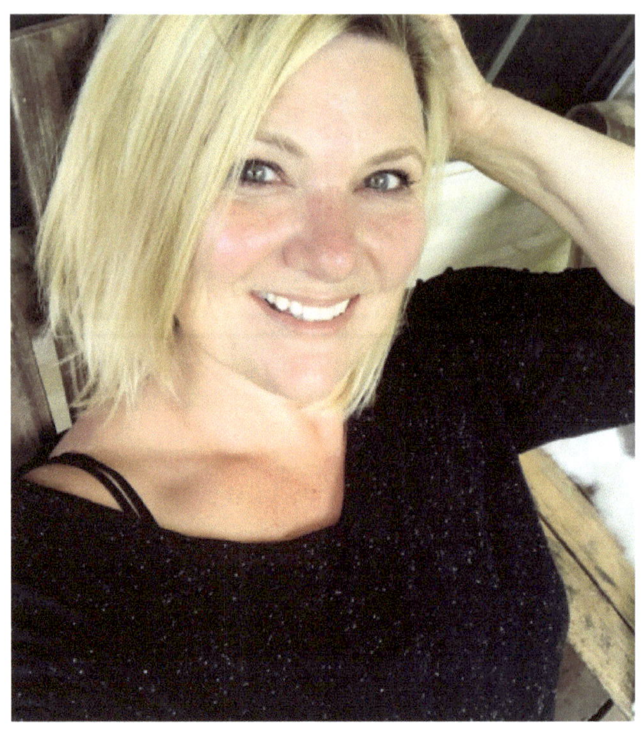

AFTER mytransformation Summer 2020

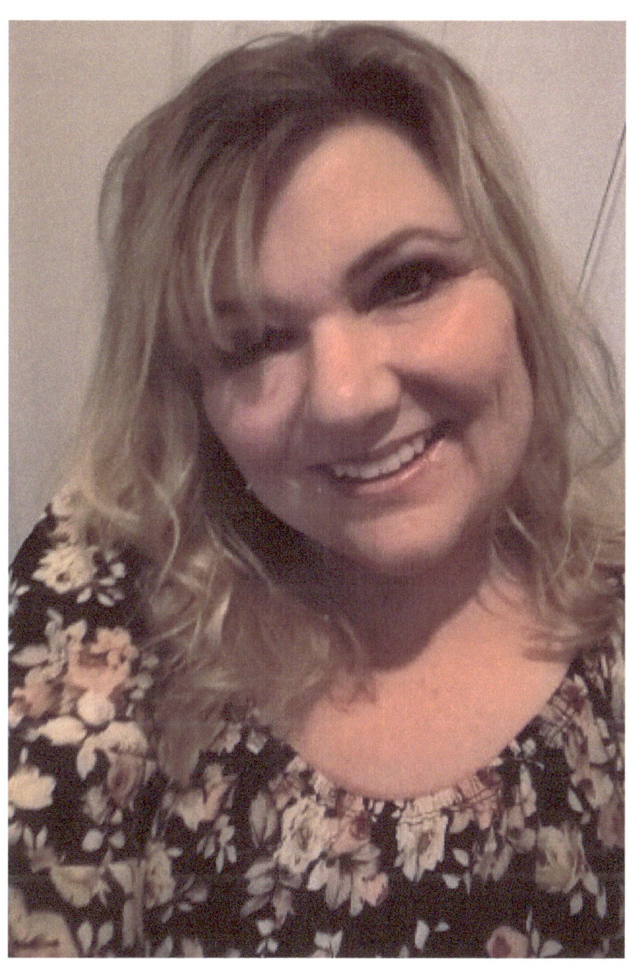

Before my transformation 2017

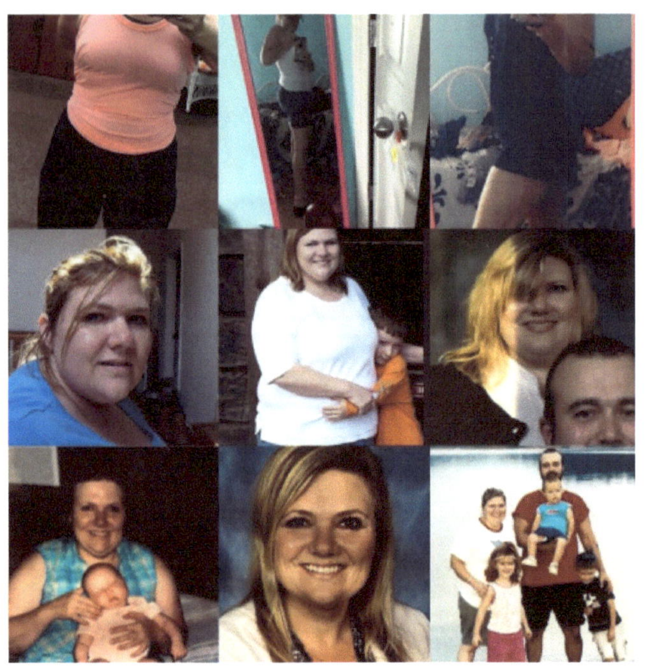